Menopause

A Positive Approach to Menopause. Diagnosing It, Identifying Symptoms and Finding Natural Treatments & Medications For An Active, Healthy Life.

Table of Contents

Introduction

Chapter 1 Menopause Signs and Symptoms

Chapter 2 Managing Your Menopause Symptoms

Chapter 3 Eat Healthy to Better Manage Your Menopause

Chapter 4 Exercises During Menopause

Chapter 5 Menopause and Your Bone Health

Chapter 6 Hormone Replacement Therapy (HRT)

Chapter 7 Self-help Relaxation Techniques

Chapter 8 Complementary Therapies and Natural Remedies

Conclusion

Introduction

This book contains proven steps and strategies on how to manage menopause. Menopause is an integral part of middle age women's life. Hot flashes, Low sex drive, weight gain, mood swings, depression, memory problem, fatigue, joint pain, fibrocystic breasts, and osteoporosis are the common symptoms and health problems during your menopause.

If you are going through the menopause and confused by conflicting advice about HRT, unsure about alternative therapies, and want to know about self-help techniques and natural remedies to deal with menopause, then good news for you is this book gives you complete solution on discovering your place in life as a middle-aged woman on her menopause.

The author of this book has consulted with health practitioners, medical experts, and menopause aged women like you to give you the best advice on staying upbeat and healthy throughout this stage of your life. The guide explains common physical and psychological symptoms and offers a holistic approach to help you manage them, including dietary and simple lifestyle changes, self-help methods, complementary therapies, natural remedies and much, much more.

☐ **Copyright 2016 by Lifestyledawn - All rights reserved.**

Chapter 1 - Menopause Signs and Symptoms

Medically speaking, menopause is the time in your life when you naturally stop having menstrual periods. The menopause is a natural part of your life and it announces the end of your fertility, meaning you are no longer fertile, unable to get pregnant and have children.

The time leading up to menopause is called perimenopause, which is a period of 12 months. During this time a woman's hormone levels begin to decrease. Menopause is not an illness; it is a natural biological process. Menopause can cause different emotional and physical symptoms of varying severity that can be disruptive to emotional health, physical energy, and sleep, and all of them can be treated.

What happens at menopause?

When a female child is born, she has about a million eggs in each ovary. At puberty roughly 300,000 eggs remain and by menopause, there are no active eggs left, thus women become infertile.

When does menopause occur?

On average, women have about 400 to 500 periods in their lifetime. As they reach the age of 35 to 40, the eggs in the ovaries decrease quickly and they ovulate (releasing the egg from the ovary) irregularly until they stop periods. Most women reach their menopause between 45 to 55 years. The average age of menopause for women is 51 to 52 years. Occasionally, menopause can occur earlier than expected because of surgery, cancer treatment or unknown causes.

The signs and symptoms of menopause start to show during the perimenopause stage. There are a variety of common symptoms of menopause and different women will show signs and symptoms differently. For some women, perimenopause stage will show very few symptoms, while others will have major symptoms that greatly affect their quality of life. Here are some common symptoms of menopause:

- Irregular periods: Menstrual cycles become shorter, longer or completely irregular, with lighter or heavier flow.

- Changes to mood and memory: Irritability, anxiety, panic attacks, mood swings, and occasional memory loss are the signs of perimenopause. Some women see menopause as signs of aging and suffer from low self-esteem or depression.

- Hot Flashes: Approximately 75% women will experience hot flashes that can lead to sweating. As estrogen levels drop in women's body, hot flashes, and sweating starts. Nighttime hot flashes are known as night sweats.

- Changes to appearance: Low estrogen levels also lead to increased rates of wrinkling, and other physical changes such as thinning hair, loss of breast fullness and increased abdominal fat.

- Mild incontinence: Some women may suffer from reduced bladder control during perimenopause and beyond, which can lead to minor urine leakage, especially when sneezing or laughing.

- Sleep disturbances or Insomnia: Approximately 4 in 10 women suffer a sleep problem, including difficulty falling or staying asleep and sleep apnea.

- Vaginal discomfort and Sexual changes: Low levels of estrogen cause vaginal dryness or decreased lubrication, which lead to painful intercourse. Also, perimenopause women have reduced sensitivity in their sexual organs because of the low blood flow to these areas.

- Fatigue or joint pain.

Chapter 2 - Managing Your Menopause Symptoms

Following are some effective self-help techniques to manage the symptoms of menopause:

Irregular or heavy periods

Irregular periods are often the first sign of the menopause. Here are tips how you can manage it:

- Gentle physical activity or heat can relieve mild period pain. For stronger pain, you need painkillers, talk to your doctor.

- Longer periods and heavy bleeding can lower your iron levels. So eat iron-rich foods, such as green leafy vegetables, lean red meat, poultry, fish and enriched whole grain bread and cereals. Take vitamin C rich foods and drinks so your body can absorb iron.

- Keep some tampons or sanitary pads with you to tackle irregular periods.

Hot Flashes

With hot flashes, you experience a feeling of heat in your chest, neck, and face. Hot flashes are usually followed by whole body sweating. They can occur without any warning, but may be brought on by stress, changes in room temperature, spicy food, alcohol or a hot caffeine-rich drink. Tips to manage it:

- Wear clothes made of natural fabrics to make yourself more comfortable and absorb moisture.

- Wear layers of clothes so you can adjust when your body temperature changes.

- Use bed sheets that you can easily throw on and off

- A cold drink can help to control the flush. So keep a glass of cold water beside your bed at night.

- Use moist wipes or water sprays to lower your skin temperature.

- Certain food and hot drinks can trigger hot flashes. So try to identify your particular trigger.

Vaginal discomfort and Sexual changes

Tips to manage it:

- Wear comfortable underwear.

- Apply a water-based lubricating jelly before sex.

- If you lose interest in sex, then talk to your partner about any worries you may have. Sex therapy or relationship counselling is also helpful.

Sleep disturbances or Insomnia

Tips to manage it:

- Physical activity and exercise help you sleep better and lower other symptoms.

- Avoid caffeine drinks such as tea, coffee or spicy foods before bed.

- If you wake during the night, get off your bed and do some mildly stimulating activity such as reading or listening to soft music until you feel sleepy again.

- Talk to your counsellor if you feel your sleep is disturbed by anxiety.

Anxiety, depression and panic attacks

Along with anxiety and depression, some women experience panic attacks for the first time at menopause.

Tips to manage it:

- Talk to your friends, family members and partner about how you are feeling. This approach will help both you and others to realize what you are going through. Talking may also help you find out the exact cause of your feelings.

- Don't think too far ahead and take each day at a time.

- Take care yourself. Relax, walk in the park, take up a hobby.

- Join a support group.

- Talk to your doctor if your feelings of anxiety and depression get worse.

Memory Loss

Tips to manage it:

- Take notes, write lists and leave them on the fridge or on the kitchen table or any other place where you will see them.

- Use your smartphone to remind you things.

- Ask people to remind you things.

- Always place your regularly used items, such as car keys, remote, glasses on the same spot.

Chapter 3 - Eat Healthy to Better Manage Your Menopause

Every woman's menopause signs and symptoms are different and how you decide to manage your menopause will depend on what symptoms you have, your age and how they affect your quality of life. There are a number of things you can do to manage your menopause, and we are going to start with a healthy eating habit.

Eat healthy

Eating healthy is a great way to manage your menopause. Before menopause, women are protected by the hormone oestrogen against a variety of diseases, such as osteoporosis, heart disease, and stroke. However, once your body starts to stop producing oestrogen, your risk of these diseases increases exponentially. Following a diet plan can help you protect against them. Low oestrogen levels also affect other parts of your body such as hair, skin and bladder.

What is the shape of your body: Apple or Pear?

With age you, your body hormones change and metabolism gradually slow down, you start to gain weight and find harder to lose it. Which part of your body accumulates weight is important for lowering your risk of heart disease. As oestrogen production lowers in your body, fat reduces around your hips and breasts and redistributes itself around the stomach. This gives your body an "Apple" shape. Various studies have shown that an apple body shape is linked with raised blood pressure, increase the risk of heart disease, type 2 diabetes and some types of cancer. Regular physical activity and a healthy diet can minimize these risks. Alternatively, if you have extra body fat stored around your hips, your body will have a "Pear" body shape, which is considered less harmful to your health.

Establish healthy eating habits:

A balanced, healthy and nutritious diet will help support general health and a healthy menopause during this time:

Eat plenty of:

- Complex carbohydrates, such as wholegrain bread, brown rice, oats to help sustain energy release.
- Legumes because they are a good source of vegetable iron and protein.
- Nuts and seeds, providing fiber, calcium and omega oils.
- Eat fresh vegetables, especially dark leafy vegetables, which provide your body micronutrients. Fresh fruits, especially potassium rich bananas to help support a healthy fluid retention. Eat at least 5 portions of fruit and vegetables daily.
- Essential fatty acids (good fats) from oily fish, such as salmon, pilchards, herring, sardines.

Eat foods rich in:

- Fiber. Eat fiber-rich vegetables, fruit and whole grains such as quinoa, bulgur wheat, brown rice, and oats. Fiber helps digestion, maintain steady blood sugar levels and lower bad cholesterol.
- Calcium for bone health
- Daily 20-minute midday sun exposure to get vitamin D, which ensures that your calcium intake is properly absorbed by the body. Vitamin D from the sun also lifts your mood and makes your productive.
- Potassium rich foods. Potassium helps to balance the sodium presence in the body and support a healthy water retention and thus help maintain a steady blood

pressure. Salmon, tuna, herring, halibut, mackerel, Swiss Chard, Brussels sprouts, broccoli, spinach, bok choy, beets, tomatoes, mushrooms, cantaloupe, avocados, figs, kiwi, coconut, almonds, Brazil nuts, yogurt, all are rich in potassium.

- Tryptophan rich foods such as sunflower seeds, sesame, milk, and eggs. Tryptophan helps to increase the production of serotonin in the body. Serotonin is known as feel good hormone and help to lift mood and promote better quality sleep.

Develop a habit of eating smaller but frequent meals throughout the day. This will help maintain steady blood sugar levels and prevent worsening of menopausal symptoms.

Drink

- Drink at least 8 glasses of filtered water to maintain body temperature and good hydration

- Freshly squeezed fruit and vegetable juice, with fiber

- Soya milk, a good source of protein, vitamin, minerals and omega-3 fatty acids.

Limit or avoid

- Lower your salt intake: Reduce the amount of salt you add when cooking to prevent high blood pressure and bloating. Use fresh ingredients when possible and cut down on processed foods.

- Reduce saturated fat or hard fat: Saturated fat affects your heart and artery health. Choose rapeseed or olive oil instead. Take health fat omega-3 from wild salmon, sardines, herrings, kippers, trout, and mackerel. Eat at least one portion of oily fish every week.

- Highly processed food, sugary foods, and junk food, which are high in salt and additives.

- Stimulants such as coffee, tea, and alcohol. These drinks produce heat and act as an obstacle to the absorption of nutrients in the body.

- Quit smoking.

Chapter 4 - Exercises During Menopause

Regular physical activity and exercise can improve and increase your strength, energy, stamina, and flexibility. Improve function of vital organs and condition of your muscles, heart and lungs. Besides these benefits, exercise can help manage many of the symptoms of menopause, including:

- Irritability, anxiety, depression
- Insomnia and sleep disturbances
- Joint pain
- Hot flashes
- Vaginal and bladder atrophy

You need a balanced program of aerobic activity, strength training, stretching and flexibility, stability and balance moves to get the benefits of physical activity.

- Aerobic exercise: Walking, running, bicycling, swimming, and dancing are all good examples of aerobic exercise. Aerobic exercises help to burn calories, which help prevent weight gain and heart disease. Many women experience both of these symptoms during menopause. If you are not used to exercising, then start slowly and combine aerobic exercise with short periods of lower-impact activities. Remember, you don't have to do 30 minutes of exercise at a time, divide your exercise time into 10-minute session and make things easy for you.

- Strength Training: According to the National Institutes of Health, muscle-building exercises are especially important for menopause age women because they help slow the normal bone loss, which can eventually lead to osteoporosis. Also, strength training help preserves lean muscle, which is another symptom in middle-aged women. But remember, you don't have to pump iron like a bodybuilder to practice strength training. A simple exercise like walking with light dumbbells can be very useful. You can join a gym or search online and watch a few strength training videos.

- Stretching and flexibility: Stretching your muscles before and after exercise is extremely important. It keeps your joints flexible and preserves your body's range of motion; both these things start to degrade as you age. You can start by gently elongate your muscles for a couple of minutes, each morning, and evening. Careful not to overextend them.

- Stability and balance move: The balance of your body start to deteriorate as you get older. So as a menopause age woman, doing exercises that improve your body's ability to stay upright and remain steady become important. To improve your balance, you can start with a simple exercise like standing on one leg for a few seconds. If necessary, balance yourself against a chair or a wall. You can also try Tai Chi. It is a slow paced, relaxing form of exercise, and great for stability and balance.

- Yoga: Dealing with menopause is stressful and activities like yoga can lower tension through low-key approaches and calm poses. Also, studies show that yoga can improve sexual function in women who are over the age of 45 years and as you know low sex drive is one of the symptoms of menopause. We will discuss more on yoga later.

How often to exercise during menopause

According to the CDC, women younger than 65 should exercise 150 minutes of moderate-intensity aerobic exercise every week. Do strength training at least twice weekly and avoid strength training two days in a row. Do 1 to 3 minutes of stretching twice daily, along with 5 minutes of balance and stability exercises every day.

Incorporating exercise into your daily life

Don't worry if you are unable to hit your exercise goal every day. Even a small amount of physical activity daily during menopause is better than none. Try to incorporate exercise into your daily life:

- Move faster when doing your housework
- Avoid driving and walk or cycle for short journeys.
- Always take the stairs instead of the elevator.
- Park further away from the superstore or office and walk the extra bit.

Chapter 5 - Menopause and Your Bone Health

It is normal for both men and women to gradually lose bone density after the age of 35, but for menopause age women, bone loss speeds up. Studies have shown that women can lose up to 20% of their bone density in the 5 to 7 years after the menopause. This situation makes postmenopausal women more at risk of weak bones (osteoporosis) and fractures.

Why?

During the menopause, the decrease in oestrogen levels causes the rapid dip in bone density. This calcium loss makes your bones weaker and thinner, especially at the wrist, the hip, and the spine. As your bones get weaker, they break more easily and you get osteoporosis. Osteoporosis is often called the 'silent disease' because it doesn't show any symptoms.

The things you should do to prevent osteoporosis

A balanced calcium-rich diet, getting enough vitamin D and regular weight-bearing activity are the best things you can do to protect yourself from osteoporosis. Following are some things you should consider:

Calcium

Milk, cheese, and yogurt are the best sources of calcium and they also absorbed easily in the body. Your aim should be to get at least 800 mg of calcium daily (3 servings). If you already had a fracture, then you may need up to 1500 mg calcium daily. Opt for low-fat milk, cheese, and yogurt if your cholesterol levels are high. Besides dairy foods, sardines, dark leafy greens like collard greens, spinach, kale, turnips, fortified cereals, fortified orange juice, fortified soymilk, and enriched grains, bread and waffles are good sources of calcium.

Remember, you also need to eat phosphorus and magnesium rich foods and get enough vitamin D to ensure that the calcium is fully absorbed and deposited in the bones. Meat, cheese, onions, garlic, and peanuts are a good source of phosphorus. Green leafy vegetables, whole grains, meat, fish, nuts, and legumes give you plenty of magnesium. Midday sun exposure and brown rice, eggs, fish oil and lentils offer vitamin D. Lastly, quit smoking to avoid osteoporosis and other diseases.

Chapter 6 - Hormone Replacement Therapy (HRT)

Hormone Replacement Therapy

HRT provides extra oestrogen to your body to keep hormone levels steady. The additional oestrogen helps relieve the symptoms caused by the fall in hormone levels – urinary discomfort, vaginal dryness, and hot flashes. It also stimulates sex drive, reduces the risk of bowel cancer, and reduce the risk of bone fractures associated with osteoporosis.

There are basically two types of HRT:

- Oestrogen on its own. This form of HRT is given to those who have their womb surgically removed (hysterectomy).

- Oestrogen given with progestogen that is very similar to the progesterone your body naturally produces. The progestogen is given to protect you from the womb cancer.

HRT is similar to the contraceptive pill, but it is not a contraceptive. HRT provides a much lower dose of oestrogen than the contraceptive pill, so they have fewer side effects.

If oestrogen is given combined with progestogen, it can be taken in two different ways:

- Sequential or cyclical HRT – with a monthly period. There are two types of HRT:
    - Monthly HRT – You take oestrogen daily and progestogen toward the end of your menstrual cycle for 12 to 14 days.
    - Three-month HRT- You take oestrogen daily and progestogen for 12 to 14 days, every 13 weeks).

- Continuous combined HRT – Period free, this HRT is recommended for women who are postmenopausal. If a woman has not had a period for a year, then she is considered as post-menopausal. Continuous HRT includes taking progestogen and oestrogen every day without a break.

Talk to your doctor and know if taking HRT is suitable for you. Taking HRT slightly raises your risk of developing the following conditions:

- Blood clots
- Ovarian cancer
- Breast cancer
- Deep vein thrombosis
- Stroke or heart disease

So if you have a history of these diseases, then your doctor may advise you on alternative treatment. Between 2000 and 2004, a large number of medical studies analyzed the effect of HRT on postmenopausal women and found a few major health problems. This statistic made some women reluctant to use HRT. However, most medical professionals agree that if HRT is used on a short-term basis (about five years), then the benefits outweigh any health risks.

How to take HRT

There are several ways HRT can be taken, including:

- A patch that you stick on your skin
- Tablets, taken by mouth
- Oestrogen gel, which is applied to the skin and absorbed

- An implant – small pellets of oestrogen are inserted under the skin of your thigh, tummy or buttock.

How long should you take HRT

HRT requirement varies among women. Usually, women take it for 2 or 3 year and others may need it for longer. Discuss with your doctor. Depending on the form of HRT and the combinations used, the directions for taking HRT also vary. It is crucial that you follow the directions on your prescription.

You should go thorough medical check-up –breast exam, blood pressure and smear test if needed. You need check-ups for each repeat prescription, about every six months. Symptoms vary when women stop taking HRT. Some experience severe menopausal symptoms and other do not experience any signs of symptoms.

Relief of Symptoms

HRT will relieve your night sweats and hot flashes first, but regardless of your dose, you may still get occasional flashes. Your sleep may improve gradually and you should see an improvement in your sleep quality within the first four weeks. Urinary symptoms and vaginal dryness may take 6 to 8 weeks to improve, depending on how severe they were.

Side effects of HRT

Though it is similar to the contraceptive pill, HRT doesn't suit all women. You may have side effects such as nausea, unexpected bleeding, breast tenderness and premenstrual syndrome-like symptoms. If your first prescription doesn't suit your body, discuss with your doctor and change the prescription. Often minor side effects can resolve on their own and you have to be patient to feel the positive effects.

Risks of HRT

HRT and the risk of breast cancer

Recent studies have shown that taking HRT slightly increase the risk of breast cancer. However, if you take HRT for less than 10 years, then the increased risk is very small.

HRT and the risk of blood clot, heart disease, and stroke

The risk of these diseases is very small, especially if HRT is taken for about five years.

If you can't use HRT

You can manage your menopausal hot flashes with healthy lifestyle changes, such as limiting caffeinated beverages and alcohol, keeping cool and practicing relaxation techniques or relaxed breathing techniques. You can use a vaginal lubricant for vaginal dryness or painful intercourse.

Chapter 7 - Self-help Relaxation Techniques

You can use self-relaxation techniques such as visual imagery, deep breathing, and progressive muscle relaxation to relieve your menopausal symptoms.

Relaxation Breathing

- Lie down on your back and relax. Keep your hands on your belly and close your eyes.

- Breathe in through your nose and notice how your stomach expands as your breath. Fill the lower chest first, then the top part of your chest and lungs.

- Hold your breath for a few seconds, relax and then breathe out. Notice how your stomach shrinks as you release all the air from your lungs.

- Relax for 5 to 10 seconds and then repeat the practice.

- Continue to practice until you fall asleep.

Doing this exercise for only five minutes daily have a significant effect on your heart rate and blood pressure.

Progressive Muscle Relaxation

This technique was developed to tackle anxiety, but it is also an effective menopause symptom reliever.

The exercise:

- Lie down on your back and gently close your eyes. This progressive muscle relaxation technique is a whole body relaxation technique. Start from your feet and progress up your body (from feet to head).

- Tense up your feet muscles for five seconds and then relax for thirty seconds.

- Tense up your calves for five seconds, and then relax for thirty seconds. One by one tense and relax your:
    - Upper legs (both thighs)
    - Abdomen and chest
    - Buttock cheeks
    - Hands
    - Upper arms
    - Your shoulders
    - Neck
    - Jaw, eye, and head

This simple progressive muscle relaxing exercise will have a calming effect on your mind, body and help manage menopause symptoms.

Visual Imagery

Along with relaxation breathing exercise, visual imagery is another effective relaxation technique to fight menopause symptoms. You have been practicing visual imagery for much of your life (daydreaming), so you don't have to learn anything. With visual imagery, you are going to put your skill to a positive use. To practice:

- Go to a quiet place where you won't be disturbed for at least 10 to 15 minutes. Now imagine a place where you once went or want to go next. This place should be both relaxing and enjoyable.

- It may be a stunning island in the middle of the Caribbean. Picture yourself walking along a beautiful, white sandy beach, with high waves and a warm breeze. Gently breathe and vividly imagine the scenario, involve all your five senses. Enjoy the moment and come back to reality when you feel you had enough.

Quiet Ears

- Lie on your back and make yourself comfortable. Close your eyes.

- Place your hands behind your head and make sure that they are loose and relaxed. Close your ear canal by placing your thumbs in your ears. Don't worry if you hear a high-pitched rushing noise because it is normal.

- Calmly listen to the sound for about 5 to 10 minutes.

- Then place your hands by your side and try to sleep.

Toe Tensing

- Lie on your back, make yourself comfortable and close your eyes

- Notice your toes (be aware of them)

- Pull all your toes back towards your face

- Gently count to ten and relax your toes, then count to ten again

- Repeat the practice for five times.

You can draw tension from the rest of your body by alternately tensing and relaxing your toes.

Chapter 8 - Complementary Therapies and Natural Remedies

Some of the extremely effective practices and methods that help relieve menopause symptoms:

Yoga

Practicing yoga is an effective weapon against menopause syndromes such as insomnia. There are many forms of yoga practices available to promote wellbeing and mind and body harmony. Hatha yoga poses and Corpse pose are best for the beginners. Here is a few Hatha yoga practice:

1. Mountain Pose or Tadasana: To practice: stand straight; keep your feet parallel and hip-width apart. Stretch your both arms overhead your head and spread your toes and fingers.

2. Bridge pose or Setu Bandhasana: The pose calms your central nervous system, reduces anxiety, and strengthens your neck, hip, and spine. To practice: lie down on your back, breathe in, lift your back and knees off the floor and then lift your heels and stand on your toes. Try to hold the pose for at least 60 seconds, but if you find it difficult then start with 30 seconds.

3. Downward facing dog or Adho Mukha Shvanasana: To practice: get down on your hands and knees. Then lift the tailbone up and bring the knees off the floor so your body creates an upside-down V shape, with the balls of your feet and your palms touching the floor.

    4. Bring your hips up and your head down. At first, keep your knees bent, and then gradually bring your heels to the floor and straighten the legs. Inhale and hold for as long as you feel comfortable.

    5. Corpse pose or Shavasana: To practice: lie flat on your back on the floor and close your eyes. Keep your legs

comfortably apart and allow your feet and knees relax. Keep your arms beside your body and one by one focus on different parts of your body. Continue to breathe and finish yoga.

Meditation

Meditation is an effective technique to relieve mental and physical stress. The practice:

- Go to a quiet place in your home, sit in a chair and keep your back straight

- Place a hand on your stomach

- Take gentle, long breaths in through the nose and out through your mouth. Focus on the sensation in your lungs as it fills up with air

- You will know the exercise is working when you are able to feel your stomach rise and fall under your hand.

One of the benefits of meditation is it help to relieve stress and anxiety.

Aromatherapy

Aromatherapy has been used for thousands of years for dealing with numerous illness, ailments and diseases. It is a safe, gentle practice, without any side effect and you can use it to help your body ease through the transition of menopause. Essential oils can be absorbed into your body in many different ways, including inhalation, ingestion or absorption through the skin and mucous membranes. Aromatherapy stimulates the brain function, act as a pain reliever, increase cognitive function, enhances mood and promote whole body healing.

Pelvic floor or Kegel exercise

If you suffer from a sensitive bladder during menopause, then practicing pelvic floor or Kegel exercise is recommended. The exercise will strengthen the muscles that support your bladder and help manage incontinence. While you are urinating, try to stop the flow of urine to find the right muscles. When you have found these muscles, practice tightening and relaxing them anytime, anywhere. You can practice this exercise when taking a bath or shower, while watching TV or while sitting on your desk at your office. Practice regularly but be careful not to overdo it.

Natural Remedies

Here are some effective natural remedies to manage your menopause symptoms

- Black Cohosh: Black cohosh is derived from a type of buttercup. Some studies show that it helps with mild hot flashes, night sweats and may lower blood pressure.

- Red Clover: Red clover contains isoflavones, which have an oestrogen-like effect in your body. Controlled trials have shown that red clover has a modest effect on lowering menopausal symptoms.

- Stinging Nettle: Nettle nourishes your postmenopausal adrenals with nettle infusion and produces enough estrogen to keep you looking and feeling healthy. Some postmenopausal women describe that stinging nettle is so nourishing and energizing that they surprisingly have a normal menstrual flow when used it regularly.

- Red ginseng: Red ginseng helps to relieve menopausal symptoms such as insomnia, hot flushes, depression, and anxiety. However, use red ginseng with caution because it has some adverse effects, such as skin eruptions, asthma, hypertension, and diarrhea.

- Motherwort: Motherwort is effective against hot flashes, mood swings and has the ability to ease heart palpitations. This herb is extremely popular with menopausal women.

- Dong Quai: Dong Quai is usually taken in as a liquid extract or capsule form and helps ease the body's hormonal transition during menopause.

- Chaste Tree Berry: For hundreds of years, chaste tree berry has been used as a supplement to treat hormonal imbalances in women. Chaste tree berry treats symptoms like hot flashes, mood swings, and depression.

- Soy: Some studies observed that food forms of soy like soy milk and tofu may be effective in reducing menopausal symptoms.

- Flaxseed, ground or oil: Flaxseed offer beneficial omega -3 fatty oils and lignans, which act as phytoestrogens and help relieve menopause symptoms. It is a natural flavonoid and has a progesterone-like an effect in the body.

- Vitamin E: Topical vitamin E oil applied directly to the vagina reduces hot flashes and improves lubrication.

Conclusion

For middle-aged women, menopause is a completely natural bodily activity. Follow the advice of this book and you don't have to worry about anything.

www.ingramcontent.com/pod-product-compliance
Lightning Source LLC
Chambersburg PA
CBHW070430190526
45169CB00003B/1486